EDUCATIONAL OUTCOMES: ASSESSMENT OF QUALITY— A COMPENDIUM OF MEASUREMENT TOOLS FOR ASSOCIATE DEGREE NURSING PROGRAMS

Carolyn F. Waltz
and
Lois H. Neuman

Editors

Pub. No. 18-2267

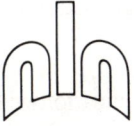

National League for Nursing • New York

Developed in conjunction with the accreditation outcomes project funded by the Helene Fuld Health Trust

Copyright © 1988 by
National League for Nursing

All rights reserved. No part of this book may be reproduced in print, or by photostatic means, or in any other manner, without the express written permission of the publisher.

Proceeds from the sale of this publication will be used for implementing the recommendations of the outcomes study.

ISBN 0-88737-433-6

Manufactured in the United States of America

Contents

Preface v
    Alan S. Trench

Foreword vii
    Sylvia E. Hart

About the Authors ix

Overview of the Compendium xi
    Sylvia E. Hart

Chapter 1 Tools for Measuring Cognitive Outcomes
    in Associate Degree Nursing Programs 1
    Lois H. Neuman and Carl H. Miller

Chapter 2 Tools for Measuring Performance Outcomes
    in Associate Degree Nursing Programs 25
    Barbara M. Sylvia and M. Dianne Bukoski

Chapter 3 Tools for Measuring Affective Outcomes
    in Associate Degree Nursing Programs 65
    Lois H. Neuman and Carl H. Miller

Selected References on Reliability and Validity 89

Preface

The Helene Fuld Health Trust has provided financial support for nursing students for nearly 20 years. Since 1969, more than $45 million have been awarded to over 400 schools of nursing. By providing funds to the National League for Nursing (NLN) for the accreditation outcomes project, the trust supported its first project that is national in scope.

The accreditation outcomes project was awarded by the trust to NLN because the League is the officially recognized accrediting body for nursing education programs. As such, NLN is committed to the assessment and recognition of high quality in nursing education programs. As a result of this project, the quality of nursing education programs will be more comprehensively and validly assessed because that quality will be determined, at least in part, by the quality of the products of those programs—the nurses who have graduated from them. Within that context, the consumer of health and nursing services will be the ultimate beneficiary.

This publication, one of several dealing with the project's findings, provides useful information about a variety of measurement tools currently being used by associate degree nurse educators. It is anticipated that this reference will be useful to those who are concerned with assessing the cognitive, affective, and performance outcomes of their students.

Alan S. Trench
Vice President
Marine Midland Bank, NA

Foreword

This publication is one of several that have resulted from NLN's Accreditation Outcomes Project. Funded by the Helene Fuld Health Trust, the project was designed to assess the state of the art in student outcomes measurement, to identify outcomes that are or should be measured, and to generate recommendations that would facilitate the inclusion of more outcome-oriented assessment in NLN's accreditation program.

This publication includes a representative sample of measurement tools submitted to project staff by associate degree nurse educators in response to the mailed survey. The document will serve as a useful reference for associate degree nurse educators as they make decisions about the outcomes and quality of programs.

Sylvia E. Hart, PhD, RN
Project Manager

About the Authors

M. Dianne Bukoski, MS, RN is an instructor at the Collingswood Nursing Center in Potomac, Maryland. Ms. Bukoski was a research associate for the project.

Sylvia E. Hart, PhD, RN is Professor and Dean at the University of Tennessee. Knoxville, College of Nursing. Dr. Hart was project manger for the Helene Fuld Health Trust Accreditation Outcomes Project.

Carl H. Miller, DNSc, RN is a professor of nursing at the University of Alabama. Dr. Miller was a research associate on the project.

Lois H. Neuman, MS, RN is professor of nursing at Prince George's College in Largo, Maryland, and is a doctoral candidate in College of Education at the University of Maryland. Ms. Neuman was a research associate for the project.

Barbara M. Sylvia, MS, RN is downstate coordinator for the RN-BSN program offered by Wilmington College, New Castle, Delaware. Ms. Sylvia is a doctoral candidate in the School of Nursing at the University of Maryland and was a research associate for the project.

Carolyn F. Waltz, PhD, RN is Professor and Coordinator for Evaluation at the University of Maryland School of Nursing. Dr. Waltz was project director for this project.

Overview of the Compendium

All measurement tools that were submitted by representatives of the associate degree nursing programs were considered for inclusion in this publication. Instruments that were highly specific to just one course in a given program were excluded because of the lack of utility of that instrument for other programs. When instruments submitted by several different schools were identical, only one such instrument was included.

The tools are presented in three categories: cognitive, performance, and affective. Within each of these categories, measurement tools are presented alphabetically by the name of the institution. The outline for each tool is as follows:

> Author
> Title
> Purpose
> Description
> Conceptual Basis
> Administration
> Scoring
> Reliability/Validity/Cost
> Contact Person

If one or more of these headings is absent for a specific tool, it is because the information was not available. Specifically, there were virtually no instruments with reliability, validity, or cost data and few tools with a reported conceptual basis. Hence, those headings are not included for most tools. All the information included for each tool was provided to project staff at the time of the mailed survey or during follow-up telephone conversations.

The references at the end of the book are provided as a guide to those who are interested in methods and procedures for establishing the reliability and validity of measurement tools.

> Sylvia E. Hart
> Project Manager

1 Tools for Measuring Cognitive Outcomes in Associate Degree Nursing Programs

Lois H. Neuman and Carl H. Miller

The tools included in this chapter are representative of those submitted by associate degree educators as samples of instruments being used to assess the cognitive outcomes of their students. Cognitive outcomes are defined as intellectual mastery or mastery of knowledge.

Author	**Bacone College**
Title	**IPR Evaluation**
Purpose	To evaluate written work.
Description	A 1-page form listing the 9 areas to be included in a process recording. Possible points are assigned to each area for a total of 10 points.
Administration	The tool is given to students as a guide to organizing the assignment.
Scoring	Each assignment has possible points. The points earned may be a part of or all the possible points. To pass, the student must receive 70 percent of the possible points. These points are averaged into the theory grade.
Contact Person	Billie Tower Chairperson Division of Health Science Bacone College Muskogee, OK 74401 (918) 683-4581

Author	**Bacone College**
Title	**Evaluation Seminar Skills Lab**
Purpose	To evaluate a student's presentation in a seminar.
Description	A one-page form that identifies five behaviors that are expected of a student when presenting a topic in a seminar class. Each behavior can be rated in a column on a weekly basis and a brief comment made.
Administration	The instructor completes the tool.
Contact Person	Billie Tower Chairperson Division of Health Science Bacone College Muskogee, OK 74401 (918) 683-4581

Author	**Cecil Community College**
Title	**Accumulated Deficiencies**
Purpose	To keep records on a student's behavior.
Description	A one-quarter page grid, with blocks labeled: week number, points, critical elements, and semester total, respectively. This form is included as part of the clinical evaluation format document.
Administration	The document is used by the faculty to record points related to the behavior of an identified student.
Scoring	Points are totaled at the end of the semester and contribute to the overall points for the course.
Contact Person	Lois Lowry Director of Nursing Cecil Community College Associate Degree Nursing Program 1000 North East Road North East, MD 21901 (301) 287-6060

Author	**Fulton Montgomery Community College**
Title	**Communication Skills Checklist**
Purpose	To present guidelines for student's communication skills.
Description	A three-page form that identifies specific behaviors as ineffective and effective during an interaction. The behaviors are listed in columns under five headings: initiating the instruction, questioning, listening, observation and problem solving. No entries are made on the handout.
Administration	The checklist is distributed to students.
Contact Person	Theresea Becker Director Fulton Montgomery Community College Johnston, NY 12095

Author	**Hutchinson Community College**
Title	**Clinical Written Work Evaluation Tool and Process Recordings Evaluation Tool**
Purpose	To evaluate written work.
Description	Two two-page tools that identify components to be evaluated for each written assignment. The components are identified under headings and are assigned points. The points are recorded for each component on the line beside each item. The final grade, date, and lines for the student's and instructor's names are on the first page.
Administration	The faculty member completes the tool.
Scoring	Each assignment reflected by these tools is graded based on 100 points. The points are assigned to the components and then totaled for a total point grade. The student must receive an average of 70 percent on written work. This grade becomes a part of the course grade. Theory and clinical grades are combined.
Contact Person	Lois Churchill Director Hutchinson Community College 1300 North Plum Street Hutchinson, KS 67501 (316) 665-3571

Author	**Kaskaskia College**
Title	**Nursing Process Form**
Purpose	To teach students to utilize nursing process components by completing a written assignment.
Description	An 11-page form. Page 1 includes the grading sheet, which lists criteria and has a space for the overall rating. Pages 2–8 contain assessment and list items for subjective data, objective data, and needs assessment. Pages 9–11 consist of a 5-column form with the labels of nursing diagnosis, short-term goals, intervention, rationale, and evaluation, respectively.
Conceptual Basis	Maslow's hierarchy of needs and Erikson's stages of development.
Administration	The student completes one for each course except the first course.
Scoring	Forms are scored as satisfactory, unsatisfactory, or incomplete. Students must receive a satisfactory grade and may repeat one time if needed to obtain a satisfactory grade.
Contact Person	Violet Draper Director Associate Degree Nursing Program Kaskaskia College Shattuc Road Centralia, IL 62801 (618) 532-1981

Author	**Kaskaskia College**
Title	**Process Recording Grading Scale and Process Recording Form**
Purpose	To evaluate the student's and patient's communication.
Description	The tool is used only in the psychiatric nursing course. It is a one-page form listing grading scale, identification of the student, date, and the patient's initials. Also included is content, possible points, points received, space for comments, total points, and the instructor's name. Specific content is listed, such as introductory data (setting, description of client, introduction of self), communication skills, and evaluation. The form consists of four columns, each headed client communication, evaluation of client, nurse communication, evaluation.
Administration	The tool is used in the clinical setting. The points on the paper are utilized only to grade the paper and are not counted as points earned in the course.
Scoring	The form indicates the possible points and points received and is converted to a satisfactory or unsatisfactory grade. Points are used as a guide to help students identify strong areas and areas that need improvement. The student must receive a satisfactory grade to pass the clinical component of the course.
Contact Person	Violet Draper Director Associate Degree Nursing Program Kaskaskia College Shattuc Road Centralia, IL 62801 (618) 532-1981

Author	**Kaskaskia College**
Title	**Follow-up of Progression**
Purpose	A record-keeping tool to perform a statistical analysis using admission test grades, course grades, and state board grades.
Description	A 1-page grid with the following headings: name, age, NLN preadmission, ACT, NLN Achievement, Basic I, Basic II, Basic III, final course grade, NLN Achievement, OB/Peds/maternal-child course grades, NLN Achievement Comprehensive Totals, course grades: 205, 206, 207, 208, State Board scores.
Administration	Students' grades are recorded.
Scoring	Information on the tool is analyzed for patterns and to evaluate the components of the program and the students' success.
Contact Person	Violet Draper Director Associate Degree Nursing Program Kaskaskia College Shattuc Road Centralia, IL 62801 (618) 532-1981

Author	**Louisiana State University at Eunice**
Title	**Guide for Writing IPR**
Purpose	To assist freshman students in writing a process recording.
Description	A one-page form. Half the page describes the information to be included on the form and the other half is the form itself. The IPR tool is divided into four columns: the patient's communication, interpretation of the patient's behavior, the nurse's communication, and evaluation of the nurse's response.
Administration	The student completes two semesters. The instructor reviews the assignment with the student at a postconference in the area of clinical work.
Scoring	The assignment is graded as acceptable or unacceptable. The student must have two acceptable scores during the semester. The grades for these assignments are part of the clinical grade.
Contact Person	Irma Andrus Head, Division of Nursing and Allied Health Louisiana State University at Eunice Box 1129 Eunice, LA 70535 (318) 457-7311

Author	**Louisiana State University at Eunice**
Title	**Care Plan**
Purpose	To provide a worksheet and an example of an acceptable care plan used throughout the nursing program except for the first semester.
Description	A five-column form and a three-page sample care plan. Headings for the form to be completed by the student are priority needs, expected outcomes, nursing actions, rationale, and evaluation. The patient's initials, diagnosis, student's name, and long-term goal are written at the top of the page.
Administration	The student submits the plan to the instructor who grades it as acceptable or unacceptable and returns it to the student.
Scoring	The student must have two acceptable plans during each semester. Once the plans are mastered, the student does not have to complete any more for that course. The grades on the care plan are part of the clinical grade.
Contact Person	Irma Andrus Head, Division of Nursing and Allied Health Lousiana State University at Eunice Box 1129 Eunice, LA 70535 (318) 457-7311

Author	Monroe Community College
Title	**Nursing Process Paper and Recording of SOAP Notes**
Purpose	To provide criteria for the grading and evaluation of written work (SOAP) in psychiatric nursing.
Description	A two-page form. The first page lists criteria and percentages that each item count toward the total score of a nursing process paper. The second page lists the evaluation criteria for the SOAP note with yes, no, and doesn't apply in columns next to the criteria.
Conceptual Basis	The nursing process.
Administration	Students complete written work based on the guidelines. The assignments are evaluated by the faculty.
Scoring	For the Nursing Process paper, 70 percent is satisfactory. The percentage score is only for feedback to the student. It is converted to a satisfactory/unsatisfactory grade, which becomes a component of the clinical grade, which is also satisfactory/unsatisfactory.
Contact Person	Helen Charron Chairperson Monroe Community College 1000 East Henrietta Road Rochester, NY 14623 (716) 424-5200

Author	Monroe Community College
Title	**Nursing Process Record—Labor and Delivery/Newborn/Postpartum**
Purpose	To present guidelines and criteria for grading written papers in the clinical area.
Description	A one-page handout providing information about the purpose, guidelines, and criteria for grading. Approved nursing diagnosis for 1984 are listed.
Conceptual Basis	The nursing process.
Administration	Part of the assignment is due prior to the clinical assignment at the preconference of the first clinical day. The second part is due after caring for the patient, following clinical experience as requested by the instructor.
Scoring	A score of 70 percent is considered satisfactory and is counted as pass/fail as part of the clinical grade. The percentages are only for feedback to students. The course grade is the theory grade but clinical components must be passed to complete the course successfully.
Contact Person	Helen Charron Chairperson Monroe Community College 1000 East Henrietta Road Rochester, NY 14623 (716) 424-5200

Author	**Motlow State Community College**
Title	**Mock Code Lab**
Purpose	To evaluate students' performance as a team during a mock code.
Description	A three-page form that identifies specific behaviors of each member of a code team. Columns for rating whether the clinical behaviors were accomplished and a brief comment line are opposite each behavior. The front sheet also identifies students on the team, evaluators, the time frame of the code, and the grade.
Conceptual Basis	Roy's adaptation model and the nursing process.
Administration	Evaluation is performed by the team of instructors teaching the course with students in the last semester of the program just before graduation.
Scoring	Clinical behaviors are rated as yes/no.
Contact Person	Betty Riddle Director Motlow State Community College Department of Nursing Education Tullahoma, TN 37388 (615) 455-8511

Author	**Motlow State Community College**
Title	**Criteria for Student Presentations**
Purpose	To present guidelines for the preparation, presentation, and evaluation of a group project.
Description	A two-page form that consists of general and specific guidelines to be used in presenting information on nursing aspects of drug therapy. Criteria for the evaluation of this group project are identified as are the points assigned to the various elements of the presentation.
Conceptual Basis	Roy's adaptation model and the nursing process.
Administration	In the second semester, first-year students present information in a group on a specific date. Evaluation is completed by the team of instructors who teach the course.
Scoring	A maximum of 50 total points can be assigned which are included as part of the grade for the course.
Contact Person	Betty Riddle Director Motlow State Community College Department of Nursing Education Tullahoma, TN 37388 (615) 455-8511

Author	Motlow State Community College
Title	**Evaluation of Teaching Learning Videotape**
Purpose	To present guidelines and a grading form for an assignment related to interviewing techniques.
Description	A 1-page form listing 10 areas used to determine the score for the videotape. Points earned are recorded next to each area on the lined portion of the form. Space for comments is provided on half the form.
Conceptual Basis	Roy's adaptation model and the nursing process.
Administration	The team of faculty members assigned to work with first-semester, first-year students views the videotapes. The whole team is then responsible for the grading.
Scoring	The assignment is worth a total of 50 points. These points, along with those earned in other assignments, collectively equal the course grade.
Contact Person	Betty Riddle Director Motlow State Community College Department of Nursing Education Tullahoma, TN 37388 (615) 455-8511

Author	New Hampshire Vocational Technical College—Stratham, Associate Degree Nursing Program
Title	**Guidelines for Patient Case Study**
Purpose	To evaluate a student's case-study paper.
Description	A 3-page form that lists all the elements to be included in a case study and assigns a point value for each section, for a total of 100 points.
Administration	This form is used for each case study developed by students. The evaluation is considered in determining a pass/fail clinical grade.
Scoring	Points are assigned to each segment of the case study, for a total of 100 available points.
Contact Person	Karen Noonan Chairperson Department of Nursing New Hampshire Vocational-Technical College 277 Portsmouth Avenue, Rte. 101 Stratham, NH 03885 (603) 772-1194

Author	**Pasadena City College**
Title	**Nursing Guidelines: Preassessment**
Purpose	To provide an example and a blank form for a written assignment in the clinical area.
Description	A two-page form that emphasizes the assessment phase of the nursing process and a preassessment phase of the identification of potential problems. An example of completed preassessments using the NCP format is provided.
Administration	Students complete the assignment in preparation for clinical assignment before going in the clinical area.
Scoring	Subjective scoring with no actual grade determined.
Contact Person	K.T. deQuerioz Chairperson Pasadena City College 1570 East Colorado Boulevard Pasadena, CA 91106 (818) 578-7323

Author	**Pasadena City College**
Title	**Directions and Guidelines for Completing the Nursing Care Study and Criteria for Grading.**
Purpose	To provide guidelines and criteria for grading a nursing care study.
Description	A one-page form that describes the requirements of assignments with point values for specific areas.
Administration	The form is given to students as a guide for writing the assignment.
Scoring	Areas are worth 4–20 points, as defined. The information is subjective. Usually points on the nursing care study are incorporated into the clinical grade, but the extent of incorporation may vary from course to course that contains clinical components.
Contact Person	K.T. deQuerioz Chairperson Pasadena City College 1570 East Colorado Boulevard Pasadena, CA 91106 (818) 578-7323

Author	**Pasadena City College**
Title	**Student's Cumulative Record of Clinical Evaluation Tool**
Purpose	To keep records of the student's midterm and final clinical evaluation scores.
Description	A one-page form on which the student's grades are recorded for all four semesters. Sixteen evaluation items are listed with boxes to record all grades including the midterm and final. The items represent the subheadings used on the clinical evaluation criteria throughout the program.
Administration	The student has a required midterm conference and may have a final conference.
Scoring	Scores (item and totals) from the CET are copied on the recording form.
Contact Person	K.T. deQuerioz Chairperson Pasadena City College 1570 East Colorado Boulevard Pasadena, CA 91106 (818) 578-7323

Author	**Wharton County Junior College**
Title	**Evaluation of Nursing Process**
Purpose	To evaluate the use of the nursing process in the clinical area.
Description	A two-page form that identifies by a word or a brief phrase items on which a student is evaluated. The items are organized under nursing process terms and each have a line to the left for ratings using a point system. The area of personal accountability is also evaluated using seven categories with behaviors in each.
Administration	The form is used to evaluate written care plans and for periodic evaluations.
Scoring	The point value for each component varies with different courses, depending on the emphasis of the course, but the total point value is 100 points. The total grade is integrated into the course. The grades from each administration of the tool during a course are averaged and then integrated into the total course grade. The percentage of the total course grade may vary for different courses.
Contact Person	Adelia Shetton Director Wharton County Junior College 911 Boling Highway Wharton, TX 77488 (409) 532-4560

Author	**Wharton County Junior College**
Title	**Abbreviated Nursing Process Form**
Purpose	To present a worksheet for developing care plans.
Description	A 1-page form divided into 20 squares and labeled with various aspects of a patient's needs, such as oxygen, nutrition, and elimination. It includes labels of pharmacology, stages of growth and development, legal ethics, and treatments. The reverse side has an outline of the human body, with directions to draw, color, or shade problems related to the patient.
Conceptual Basis	Maslow's hierarchy of needs and Erikson's stages of development.
Administration	The students complete the form using the data collected. They go out the day before to assess their clients. The evening before the clinical course, they fill out the abbreviated nursing process and hand it to the instructor at the beginning of the clinical day.
Scoring	The form is graded using the grading scale criteria for evaluation of the nursing process in the clinical area (psychomotor) of the clinical evaluation tool. The point value varies with different courses, depending on the emphasis of the course. The clinical evaluation grades are then integrated into the total grade; however, the percentage of the total course grade varies for different courses.
Contact Person	Adelia Shetton Director Wharton County Junior College 911 Boling Highway Wharton, TX 77488 (409) 532-4560

2 Tools for Measuring Performance Outcomes in Associate Degree Nursing Programs

Barbara M. Sylvia and M. Dianne Bukoski

This chapter includes a collection of measurement tools being used by associate degree nurse educators to measure the clinical performance of students and graduates of associate degree nursing programs. Performance is broadly defined as the functioning of a nursing student or graduate in the clinical setting for the purpose of meeting the health needs of clients through the direct and indirect use of the nursing process. Specific dimensions of performance include the following:

1. *Guiding and working with others in a supportive growth-promoting manner as all work to meet the health needs of clients.*

2. *Assessing, planning, and evaluating nursing care directed toward meeting the health needs of clients.*

3. *Performing skills required to meet the health needs of clients.*

4. *Teaching clients and family members how to meet their health needs better.*

5. *Communicating with clients.*

6. *Developing and maintaining personal growth.*

The performance tools submitted by the schools of nursing are predominately broad, encompassing many or all the listed dimensions of performance. The majority of the measurement tools measure performance from a broad perspective, often at the completion of a nursing course containing a clinical component. The remainder measure more discrete dimensions of performance, including process-recording forms, nursing care plans, specific components of nursing-process measurement tools, anecdotal forms, and skills checklists.

Author	**Alfred State College**
Title	**Clinical Evaluation Tool**
Purpose	For the instructor to evaluate a student's performance and for the student to use as a guide to clinical performance.
Description	Each of the four tools is constructed in the same format but the four show a progression through the nursing courses. An explanation of the evaluation process and a key for grading are on the first page. The next pages identify the critical behaviors that have been derived from the course objectives and relate to the roles of the nurse, as identified in the NLN statement of Associate Degree Competencies. Columns for grading performance at the midterm and final are next to each of the identified behaviors. The final page is for written midterm and final summaries and signatures.
Conceptual Basis	Utilization of the nursing process to meet human needs, according to the theories of Maslow and Erikson through the role of the nurse as identified in the NLN Statement of Associate Degree Competencies.
Administration	The instructor completes the tool at the midterm and the final. At the midterm conference, the instructor rates the student as satisfactory, on clinical probation for needing improvement, or unsatisfactory. Written comments are also given to the student in this formative evaluation. By the final evaluation at the end of the course, the student receives a summative evaluation and is expected to have achieved all critical behaviors satisfactorily. The faculty are moving in the direction of giving 2½-hour clinical performance examinations on a one-to-one basis as a diagnostic tool midpoint in the fourth semester
Scoring	At the midterm, there is a three-point rating system; at the final, only two— satisfactory and unsatisfactory. The behaviors for the terms are identified on each tool. Theory and clinical work are one grade. The grade includes written examinations, quizzes, written assignments, a skills

lab, and the final examination. If a student is unsatisfactory in the clinical work, the student receives an F grade.

Contact Person Marilyn Lusk
Nursing Department
Alfred State College
Alfred, NY 14802
(607) 587-3695

Author	**Arizona Western College**
Title	**Clinical Evaluation**
Purpose	To evaluate the clinical performance of freshman nursing students.
Description	Competencies are listed for each of 11 objectives and are rated as safe or unsafe at the midterm and final. Space is provided for narrative comments and signatures.
Conceptual Basis	Orem's theory of nursing.
Administration	The student receives a copy of the tool at the beginning of the course and meets weekly with the instructor. The instructor makes weekly anecdotal records on a separate form and includes that information when completing the midterm and final evaluations. The student completes the tool as a means of self-evaluation in later courses.
Scoring	Each competence needs to be safe for each objective to be achieved safely by the end of the semester. If any objective is rated unsafe, the student fails the clinical part. If a student fails the clinical work but passes theory, a D grade is given. If both theory and clinical work are failed, a grade of F is given. A computerized grading program is available to each instructor.
Contact Person	Karen Monks Chairperson Arizona Western College Box 929 Yuma, AZ 85364 (602) 726-1000

Author	**Belmont College**
Title	**Clinical Evaluation Tool**
Purpose	To evaluate the performance of freshman associate degree nursing students.
Description	A guide for use in clinical practice that lists the 25 competencies with 11 unlabeled columns and 1 column labeled "total" adjacent to the competencies. The evaluation tool lists the same 25 competencies in a 5-page form. It also has instructions, the method of evaluation, the definition of ratings and terms, and categories. Section A contains 25 competencies under 5 headings to be rated in the adjacent columns using a 4-point scale. Space for comments is provided beside each competence. Section B contains space for the grade for 2 care plans that the student selects to be evaluated from all the care plans completed during the clinical experience. The last page has designated spaces for signatures, grades, and dates for Rotation I and Rotation II.
Conceptual Basis	Roy's adaptation theory.
Administration	Formal evaluation generally occurs in the last two weeks of each rotation. The instructor completes the form and the student signs it after the evaluation conference.
Scoring	Section A is graded on a 50-point scale, with a student receiving 0–2.0 points for each of the 25 competencies. To pass the course, the student must have a total of 37.5 points in Section A. Section B is completed for each rotation. A zero in any competence at the end of a rotation will result in a zero for section A. Categories of ratings for competencies on Section A: above average = 2.0 points, average = 1.5 points, below average = 1.0 points, and unsatisfactory = 0 points. Section B is graded on a 50-point scale calculated from accumulated points on the Nursing Care Plan. For the course letter grade, Section A = 50 points possible and Section B = 50 points possible; total points = 100. A = 94–100 points, B = 85–93 points, C = 75–84 points, D = 74–65 points, and F = 64–0 points. Grades are

hand-tabulated. Theory and clinical grades are separate. Passing is C or 75 percent. Failure involves suspension from the course, but readmission is permitted the next year.

Contact Person Dr. Anna Hite
Dean
Belmont College
1900 Belmont Boulevard
Nashville, TN 37203
(615) 385-6436

Author	**Cecil Community College**
Title	**Care Plan Checklist**
Purpose	To provide a checklist and grade-point allocation.
Description	A four-page document that identifies the point allocation for identified requirements and provides space for identification of deficiencies and competencies.
Conceptual Basis	The nursing process.
Administration	Used for writing and grading care plans.
Scoring	The assignment counts as a percentage of the grade for each level. Points for components of the assignment are detailed.
Contact Person	Lois Lowry Director of Nursing Cecil Community College Associate Degree Nursing Program 100 North East Road North East, MD 21901 (301) 287-6060

Author	**Central Carolina Community College Associate Degree Nursing Program**
Title	**Student Practicum Checklist**
Purpose	To evaluate the clinical performance of students.
Description	A six-page evaluation tool containing lists of expected behaviors organized under five categories of competence: applying management theories, implementing effective leadership, coordinating groups, planning and implementing change, and working in organizations. Each behavior is graded A–F according to specific grading guidelines. Lines for narrative comment are provided, as well as a small space to record other elements considered in the course grade, such as pre- and postconference preparation and participation, attendance, and self-evaluations. The last page provides space for the instructor's and student's comments, a final grade, and signatures.
Administration	Self-administered by students.
Scoring	Used by students to make a personal assessment of their progress.
Contact Person	Gloria N. Peele Nursing Program Central Carolina Community College 530 Carthage Street Sanford, NC 27330 (919) 774-9516

Author	Clatsop Community College
Title	Clinical Evaluation I and II
Purpose	To evaluate the student's clinical performance in first- and second-year courses.
Description	These two tools are similar and both are used throughout the year. The first page contains the legend for clinical grading: grades A–F. There is space for narrative summaries at the midterm and final, signatures, and grades for various components of the course. The rest of the tool (six pages) lists clinical objectives under an organizing framework of roles and specific competencies that are rated weekly. The program quarter in which the competence is expected to be achieved is listed in a column next to the competence. Columns for weekly ratings using the key S for satisfactory, N for needs improvement, and U for unsatisfactory are beside each competence. A section of psychomotor skills according to each level completes the items to be rated. A comment section is on each page.
Conceptual Basis	The NLN competencies of an associate degree graduate.
Administration	The instructor completes the tool and holds a midterm and final conference with the student. Depending on his or her ability, the student may use the tool as a means of self-evaluation.
Scoring	Definitions for the rating scale are listed on the form. A score of A (91–100 percent) indicates above average performance and complete preparation; B (83–90 percent), average performance and preparation; C (75–82 percent), meets safety standards; D (68–74 percent), failure to meet standards for preparation and practice; and F (0–67 percent), unsafe performance. To pass the clinical course, the student must receive a C or better. The student may not progress to the next level if the clinical part is not satisfactory. If the student fails, he or she may repeat the clinical part and must audit theory. The grades are recorded by hand.
Contact Person	Karen Burke Clatsop Community College Astoria, OR 97103 (503) 325-0910

Author	Corning Community College, Associate Degree Nursing Program
Title	Terminal Behaviors
Purpose	To evaluate the student's clinical performance.
Description	A five-page evaluation tool containing a list of competencies based upon the NLN assumptions basic to the cope of practice. These competencies are organized under five categories: (1) role as a provider of care, (2) communicator, (3) patient/client teacher, (4) manager of client care, and (5) member of the profession of nursing. Columns appear to the right of the competencies to designate the level of performance as satisfactory, unsatisfactory, or needs improvement at the midterm and the end of course. Space is provided on the last page for comments.
Conceptual Basis	Role theory.
Administration	Faculty complete the tool at the midterm and the end of the last two nursing courses. No space is provided for the student's comments or for the faculty's or student's signatures.
Scoring	Satisfactory, unsatisfactory, or needs improvement is determined for each competency identified. It is expected that each competence will be evaluated as satisfactory by the end of the course.
Contact Person	Dr. Anita Ogden Chairperson Division of Nursing Education Corning Community College Spencer Hill Road Corning, NY 14830 (607) 962-9241

Author	**Dyersburg State Community College**
Title	**Clinical Evaluation Tool**
Purpose	For the student and instructor to evaluate the student's clinical performance.
Description	A 9-page form on which 87 behaviors are identified under 18 different areas. These behaviors are rated satisfactory or unsatisfactory in the columns next to each behavior. Comments/examples are written to validate the ratings. The teacher's and student's final comments are on the last page. The form is a self-evaluation tool, used in conjunction with the instructor's anecdotal notes for evaluation conferences.
Conceptual Basis	Stress-adaption theory.
Administration	The student uses the tool to write a self-evaluation at the midterm and final. The instructor writes anecdotal notes. Both the student's self-evaluation and the anecdotal notes are used for the clinical evaluation. Areas for improvement are noted during the evaluations. Unsatisfactory performance is noted in the anecdotal comments and discussed with the student and the level coordinator. Patterns of unsatisfactory performance are rated as such on the final evaluation. Final comments by the student and instructor are put on a permanent copy of the tool and kept by the instructor and retained in the student's nursing file.
Scoring	Students receive a satisfactory (S) or unsatisfactory (U) clinical grade, but they must get a satisfactory clinical grade to pass the course. To achieve a satisfactory clinical grade for the 87 listed behaviors, the student may not have more than 9 behaviors rated unsatisfactory.
Contact Person	Peggy Pendergrast Chairperson Dyersburg State Community College PO Box 648 Dyersburg, TN 38024 (901) 285-6910

Author	**Edison Community College**
Title	**Freshman Clinical Evaluation**
Purpose	To evaluate the clinical performance of freshman students.
Description	A seven-page tool. The first five pages identify nursing skills (psychomotor) and behaviors (judgement and responsibilities) that are rated on a three-point checklist. Space for comments on each item is in a third column. The last two pages are for narrative comments on course requirements and major areas of weaknesses and strengths. Lines for final grades and signatures are also on the last page.
Administration	Both the student and the instructor complete the first five pages, and the student completes the last two pages, which are for self-evaluation. The tool is completed at the midterm if the student is having difficulties and then experiences are planned accordingly. Otherwise, the written evaluation is completed at the end of the term.
Scoring	The ratings for the checklist are above average, average, and below average. An overall determination is made at the final evaluation. The student must receive a satisfactory grade to pass the course (50 percent of the scores being above average or average). The theory grade is recorded. If the student receives an unsatisfacory grade, an F is recorded, and the course may be repeated. The grades are tabulated in the school's computer center.
Contact Person	Margaret N. Anfinsen Head, Department of Allied Health Studies Edison Community College 8099 College Parkway, S.W. PO Box 06210 Ft. Myers, FL 33906 (813) 489-9239

Author	**Edna M. Clark School of Nursing**
Title	**Clinical Evaluation**
Purpose	To evaluate the clinical performance of sophomore nursing students.
Description	Modified from a generic tool, this seven-page checklist and comment form is used to identify behavioral objectives under three major headings: correlation of theory/clinical, utilization of the nursing process, and professional development. A checklist for rating behaviors on a five-point scale is beside each item, and space for comments is under each section. The final page is for a clinical summary, the student's comments, clinical grades, and signatures.
Conceptual Basis	The nursing process.
Administration	The student receives a copy of the tool at the beginning of the course and uses it for self-evaluation. The instructors rate comments after each rotation. Each instructor uses a different-colored pen.
Scoring	The rating scale is defined on the tool with behavioral statements using the following terms: outstanding (OS), above average (AA), average (AV), minimal (M), unsatisfactory (US), and not applicable (NA). The clinical grade is pass/fail. Students are expected to achieve the objectives at the minimal level. If any objectives are rated unsatisfactory, the student receives an F in clinical and does not pass the course. If the student passes the course, the theory grade is recorded.
Contact Person	Joan Kney Director Edna M. Clark School of Nursing Presbyterian Hospital 617 West 168th Street New York, NY 10032 (212) 305-2749

Author	**Felician College**
Title	**Clinical Evaluation Tool**
Purpose	To evaluate clinical performance in first and second year nursing courses.
Description	These four tools, one for each level or course, are all constructed in the same way. The first page contains an explanation of the criteria for evaluation, the definition of terms, and space for the student's signature, which indicates that the student has reviewed the tool. The following pages list the 9 through 11 major clinical objectives for each course (derived form the program and course objectives), columns for rating the student satisfactory or unsatisfactory, and space for written comments under each objective. The last page is for the instructor's and student's summary comments.
Conceptual Basis	Orem's theory of nursing.
Administration	The student receives a copy on the first day of the course, signs it, and returns it to the instructor. The student and the instructor meet weekly to discuss the student's progress. The instructor completes the tool at the end of the course and holds a final evaluation conference with the student.
Scoring	A two-level rating scale is used: S = satisfactory and U = unsatisfactory. The student must receive an S rating on each component of the clinical objectives at the final evaluation to pass the course. If the ratings are unsatisfactory at the final evaluation, the student receives an F.
Contact Person	Joan Murko Interim Director Department of Nursing ADN Department, Felician College 260 South Main Street Lodi, NJ 07644 (201) 778-1190

Author	Galveston College Associate Degree Nursing Program
Title	**Introduction to Nursing**
Purpose	To evaluate the clinical performance of beginning nursing students.
Description	An eight-page tool on which clinical objectives are described under six headings and rated as satisfactory or unsatisfactory at the mid-term and final using a checklist. The objectives are described under nursing accountability, nursing process (four steps), and documentation. The activities needed to fulfill the requirements for written assignments are listed under documentation. A line for comments is next to each item to be rated. The last page contains space for student's and faculty member's summary comments and signatures. Starred items are critical incidents.
Conceptual Basis	The nursing process.
Administration	The faculty members complete the tool at the midterm and final evaluations. The student may comment and is expected to identify learning goals.
Scoring	Items are rated as satisfactory or unsatisfactory. Starred items must be achieved satisfactorily. The theory grade appears on the transcript. If the student fails, he or she may repeat the course when it is offered, provided that the student has not failed any other clinical course.
Contact Person	Nancy Stewart Assistant Dean, Health Galveston College 4015 Avenue Q Galveston, TX 77550 (409) 763-6551

Author	**Gloucester County College, Associate Degree Nursing Program**
Title	**Clinical Evaluation Tool**
Purpose	To perform clinical evaluations.
Description	A seven-page evaluation tool listing six course objectives with specific acceptable and unacceptable criteria identified for each. Space is provided for checking either the satisfactory or unsatisfactory behavior and for comments. On the last page, there is space for recording the student's strengths and weaknesses and for the student's and instructor's signatures.
Scoring	Students are rated on each course objective according to criteria as either satisfactory or unsatisfactory. To pass the course, the student must receive an S for each objective.
Contact Person	Lucy Stetta Chairperson Nursing Program Gloucester County College Deptford Township Sewell, NJ 08080 (609) 468-5000

Author	**Hutchinson Community College**
Title	**Clinical Evaluation Tool**
Purpose	To provide a basis for more objectivity in the evaluation process.
Description	Four tools on which behavioral components identified under each course objective serve as a guide for the behaviors that are necessary to meet each objective. Each course objective is on a different page. Critical behaviors are identified with an asterisk. The course objectives focus on the nursing process and communication. The behavioral components are listed under the objective. The other half of the page is for anecdotal comments. A last page is for summary evaluations in which dates, the grade, comments, and signatures are recorded.
Administration	The tool is used by both the faculty member and the student and is passed back and forth for weekly evaluations. Both the faculty member and the student record anecdotal notes that must include the student's effort and the effect of the student's performance. By the end of the semester, each behavioral component should be addressed once. Each course objective must be addressed weekly in the first-level course and then as required. The student identifies the behavioral component when writing the narrative. Formal clinical evaluation conferences take place at least two times a semester for the first level; three times, for Nursing II and III; and two times, for Nursing IV if the student is progressing satisfactorily. The signatures of both the faculty member and the student indicate that a particular conference was held. The student may write comments. The student's performance of critical behaviors is described by the faculty member. Students may record anecdotes of these behaviors if they desire in Nursing II and III. In Nursing IV, the faculty member documents the student's behaviors related to the nursing process and the student is required to document those behaviors identified by an asterisk.

Scoring Grades are satisfactory/unsatisfactory and are recorded at the conference time. The final grade includes both hospital and nursing home experience, with greater emphasis placed on performance at the end of the semester in the Nursing I course. A U (unsatisfactory) in either setting constitutes failure. Consistent progress is emphasized within each rotation in other levels. Final clinical grades in Nursing II and above also include satisfactory grades on written work. If the student receives an unsatisfactory grade, the student may repeat the course. Theory and clinical grades are combined.

Contact Person Lois Churchill
Director
Hutchinson Community College
1300 North Plum Street
Hutchinson, KS 67501
(316) 665-3571

Author	**Indiana Vocational Technical College—Region 4**
Title	**Student Clinical Evaluation**
Purpose	To evaluate the clinical performance of upper-level students.
Description	A seven-page tool on which expected behaviors of students are identified and organized within five role categories: the nurse as provider, teacher, manager, communicator, and professional. The roles are assigned weights, as are each section and behavior within the role. Columns to record midterm and final grades on a five-point scale and a small space for comments are beside each item. Items with asterisks denote critical objectives. A larger space for comments and lines for signatures and grades are on the sixth page. The grading system, with different weights as the student progresses through the course, is explained on the last page.
Administration	The student is given a copy of the tool at the beginning of the course. The instructor reviews the tool weekly with the student for formative evaluation. There is a summative evaluation at the midterm and the final, with grades averaged for the final evaluation.
Scoring	A new scoring scale from 1 (low) to 5 (high) was recently instituted. The points are added up for all the behaviors under a given role, averaged, and then multiplied by the percentage allotted to the role. The five sections are then totaled for the final grade. Theory and clinical grades are separate. If the student fails the clinical part, he or she may repeat it. Theory may also be repeated, and the student has the option of having the higher theory grade recorded. Grades are hand-tabulated in the department.
Contact Person	Ruth Chastin Director Indiana Vocational Technical College— Region 4 3208 Ross Road Box 6299 Lafayette, IN 47903 (317) 423-5508

Author	**Iowa Central Community College Department of Nursing**
Title	**Selected Clinical Review**
Purpose	To evaluate the student's clinical performance.
Description	Three general objectives serve as the headings for 23–25 specific objectives on each form: assessment and primary nursing care, implementation of patient care, and personal and professional development. Each objective is further delineated by four sets of specific statements of behavior related to that objective, which reflect a value rating on a four-point scale. The four sets of behavioral statements are boxed off and have a column for checking off the current statement as it applies to the student's performance. The last page is a proficiency record summary sheet, with columns to record points earned according to objectives, rotations, and a grading scale.
Administration	For each rotation, the instructor rates the student's performance and places the numerical rating in the appropriate box.
Scoring	Each behavioral item is rated and given a numerical rating of 0–4 at the end of each clinical rotation during the course. Ratings are then summed and converted to a percentage point that constitutes the clinical grade. The clinical grade and theory grade are differentially weighted and then combined to derive the course grade. The student must pass both the theory and clinical parts to pass the course.
Contact Person	Delores Kollasch Head, Department of Nursing Iowa Central Community College 330 Avenue M Fort Dodge, IA 50588 (515) 576-7201

Author	Ira D. Pruitt School of Nursing, Livingston University
Title	Student's Evaluation of Achievement of Level I Objectives
Purpose	To help the student in analyzing goal achievement upon completion of a clinical course and to assist the faculty to identify the student's strengths and weaknesses.
Description	Expected clinical behaviors are described under five areas: nursing process, interpersonal skills, communication skills, team member, and current practice trends. The student is asked to rate how well he or she has achieved the objectives. Formative evaluations are done weekly; summative evaluations are done at the end of each component.
Conceptual Basis	The nursing process.
Administration	The student completes the tool and turns it in to the adviser 24 hours before the evaluation conference at the end of each component. The evaluations by both the instructor and the student are discussed; both sign the final evaluation form.
Scoring	The rating scale for the behaviors is satisfactory or unsatisfactory. Theory and clinical are one grade. A minimum grade of C in theory and a satisfactory grade in clinical are required to pass the course. If the student fails the clinical part, he or she fails the course but may repeat it.
Contact Person	Sylvia Homan Director Ira D. Pruitt Division of Nursing Livingston University Livingston, AL 35470 (205) 652-9661

Author	**Junior College of Albany, Associate Degree Nursing Program**
Title	**Skills Performance Criteria**
Purpose	To test the psychomotor performance of students.
Description	This tool is a sample of a college laboratory criterion-referenced performance test. Three skills are identified, and criteria are listed under each. Points are assigned to each criterion. The skills identified on the sample provided are irrigation of bladder via foley catheter, breast self-examination, and advanced wound dressing.
Administration	The skills-performance test is administered at the end of the term.
Scoring	Points assigned to each criterion are tallied. The student must receive 70 percent to pass the clinical portion of the course.
Contact Person	Joan Maguire Chairperson Nursing Program Junior College of Albany 140 New Scotland Avenue Albany, NY 12205 (518) 445-1734

Author	Lincoln Memorial University
Title	Clinical Evaluation Tool
Purpose	To evaluate the student's performance in the on-campus laboratory and in the clinical setting.
Description	A six-page form with columns for ratings and comments next to statements of student's behaviors in relation to the role functions of the associate degree nurse on entry into practice. Specific behaviors are identified under each role, and one page is devoted to a list of the technical skills that the student should practice. A key indicates that critical behaviors are starred (but these are not on the form). A satisfactory/unsatisfactory scale is used. An additional form contains the asterisk beside critical behaviors to show progress through the program. Different behaviors have an asterisk at different points in the program. Skills change each term, with some skills identified as critical and therefore required to pass the course.
Conceptual Basis	Competencies of the associate degree nurse and the nursing process.
Administration	The evaluative comments may be anecdotal or by delineation of areas of strength, weakness, and so on. The instructor rates behaviors as satisfactory, unsatisfactory, or not observed. A rating must have evaluative comments.
Scoring	The rating scale is as follows: S = satisfactory—objective met, U = unsatisfactory—objective not met, NA = non applicable, and NO = not observed.
	All skills for the campus laboratory must be performed satisfactorily, and critical objectives must be met satisfactorily by the end of the quarter. Also 80 percent of the non critical objectives must be achieved by the end of the quarter. Students must have an S in clinical to pass the course, but the clinical grade of S or U is not calculated in the final course grade. The final course grade is the theory grade.
Contact Person	Nancy Moody, Chairperson Lincoln Memorial University Harrogate, TN 37752 (615) 869-3611

Author	**Maryville College**
Title	**Clinical Evaluation Tool**
Purpose	To evaluate the student's performance.
Description	A seven-page form, six pages of which describe clinical objectives and critical behaviors for each objective. The objectives are organized under nursing process, technical skills, teaching, communication, and growth and accountability. A pass/fail checklist format for rating is next to each critical behavior, as well as a brief space for making comments. The front page is a narrative format, with lines for signatures and dates. The tool is modified slightly for each course to reflect the particular content of the course. The faculty is in the process of revising the tool.
Administration	The student receives a copy at the beginning of the course and completes the tool, as does the instructor at the final evaluation. The student receives a narrative evaluation at the midterm. The evaluations are kept on file for three years.
Scoring	A pass/fail checklist is used for rating. Students must complete all critical behaviors satisfactorily, but an instructor may deem a course-critical objective unavailable during a rotation. The theory and clinical parts are separate, but if the student fails either, he or she must repeat the entire course.
Contact Person	Connie Koch Director Maryville College 13550 Conway Road St. Louis, MO 63141 (314) 576-9435

Author	Mitchell Community College
Title	**Fundamentals of Nursing, Clinical Objectives and Clinical Evaluation**
Purpose	To evaluate the student's clinical performance in a fundamentals of nursing course.
Description	Eight main objectives provide the framework for identifying expected clinical competencies. The competencies under objectives 1–4 and 8 are rated by checking satisfactory or unsatisfactory on a line below the statement. Brief comments also may be made. A skill objective is rated by recording the date on which the skill is satisfactorily completed in the clinical portion. Other objectives that are related to psychomotor skills are rated by recording dates of satisfactory completion in the laboratory, as well as in the clinical area. Starred items are critical and are to be achieved satisfactorily. The last page is for a summary evaluation and signatures. The student may write comments, if he or she desires. This tool also has a page that explains the evaluation process and pages that list other requirements for the clinical area.
Administration	Students get copies of the evaluation tool and the syllabus at the beginning of each course. The instructor does a formative evaluation each week using anecdotal notes; the student signs the evaluation, which is attached to the clinical tool at the end of each quarter. The midterm evaluation is a conference for which no grade is given; emphasis is placed on identifying the student's strengths and weaknesses. The final evaluation is summative; the student receives a grade of satisfactory or unsatisfactory. The final evaluation is kept on file for three years, and the student may request a copy.
Scoring	A satisfactory/unsatisfactory rating scale is used. An unsatisfactory in the clinical area means failure of the course. The student may repeat the same course twice, but he or she must audit the nursing course preceding it. Since courses are offered only once a year, it may be a year or more before

	the student is able to repeat it. Theory and clinical grades are recorded on the transcript as one grade but are kept separate in the grade book.
Contact Person	Irene Henline Director Mitchell Community College West Broad Street Statesville, NC 28677 (704) 878-3200

Author	**Motlow State Community College**
Title	**Clinical Competencies**
Purpose	To evaluate the student's clinical performance of psychomotor skills.
Description	A one-sheet checklist listing psychomotor skills that are checked off according to set dates on the form. A small space for comments is available.
Conceptual Basis	Roy's adaptation model and the nursing process.
Administration	The clinical instructor evaluates the student's skills twice in each unit. Students are responsible for knowing all psychomotor skills. Their competence is demonstrated by their randomly selecting one skill and performing it successfully.
Scoring	On a pass/fail basis, with a pass score required to pass the course.
Contact Person	Betty Riddle Director Motlow State Community College Department of Nursing Education Tullahoma, TN 37388 (615) 455-8511

Author	**New Hampshire Technical Institute, Division of Nursing, Associate Degree Program**
Title	**Student Clinical Evaluation**
Purpose	To evaluate the student's performance in a course with a clinical component.
Description	A five-page form that identifies eight objectives for the student's clinical performance and briefly lists more specific behaviors under each objective. Columns for rating behaviors according to pass or nonpass are beside each section, and one page for summary comments is at the end. The front page has lines for identifying course dates, attendance, signatures, grades, and an educational diagnosis of the student. The nursing process, communication, teaching plan, and legal/ethical areas are the focus of the specific objectives.
Administration	The instructor and student review the form at midpoint of the course. At the end of the course, the instructor rates the student's performance and reviews the results with the student.
Scoring	All objectives and behaviors are rated as pass (P) and nonpass (NP). By the end of the course, the student must pass all the clinical objectives in order to pass.
Contact Person	Joyce Blood New Hampshire Technical Institute Fan Road Concord, NH 03301 (603) 225-1800

Author	New Mexico Junior College
Title	Evaluation Form
Purpose	To evaluate the student's clinical performance.
Description	Each of the three tools uses the same format. The cover sheet includes final grades and comments, identification information, and places for signatures. A guide explains the evaluation procedure and the student's responsibilites for self-evaluation. The instructor's responsibilities in assessing physical or emotional hazards are also explained. The guide lists behavioral expectations categorized as communication or interpersonal relationships, assessment, planning, intervention, evaluation, and personal and professional performance. A seventh category, leadership and management, appears on one form. These behavioral expectations or criteria are given values that are totaled for the final grade.
Administration	The student completes the self-evaluation and the instructor completes the evaluation of the student. Both evaluations are discussed at the midterm to determine areas that need improvement.
Scoring	A grade of pass/fail is assigned at the end of the term. Each behavior/criterion is given a percentage value. The student must achieve a grade of 75 percent for each category. The percentage is determined by calculating the percentage of criteria met out of the total number of criteria.
Contact Person	Joyce Gombar Chairperson New Mexico Junior College 5317 Lovington Highway Hobbs, NM 88240 (505) 392-4510

Author	Northern Oklahoma College Associate Degree Program
Title	**Clinical Nursing Evaluation Tool**
Purpose	To evaluate the student's performance in courses with a clinical component.
Description	A six-page form of which the top sheet is a clinical performance summary sheet. The expected clinical behaviors of students are identified under three main categories: nursing process, communication, and professional behaviors. Space for comments or rationale is allotted on each page.
Conceptual Basis	The nursing process and Maslow's hierarchy of needs.
Administration	Determined each semester by faculty for the course. The tool is typically administered at or near the end of the course, but since the faculty members make the decision, it may be administered various times during the course.
Scoring	Not all items may be rated during the course, but all are rated at the end of the course. Each behavior is weighted by the faculty according to its importance in the course. Each item is rated on a percentage or point system.
Contact Person	Delphine Jewell Chairperson Northern Oklahoma College 1220 East Grand Tonkawa, OK 74653 (405) 628-2581

Author	Piedmont Virginia Community College Program for Nursing
Title	Clinical Competencies and Summative Clinical Evaluation Form
Purpose	To evaluate the student's clinical performance.
Description	A form on which clinical competencies are identified according to 3 general areas—nursing process, wellness-illness, and accountability—with varying number of behavioral items under each category. Adjacent to the behavioral items are 17 unlabeled columns. Critical competencies are starred. The last page is for the student's self-evaluation through written comments and the faculty member's comments and recommendations.
Conceptual Basis	The nursing process, wellness-illness continuum, and accountability.
Administration	The students are given the clinical evaluation tool at the beginning of the course to use as a guide to their clinical performance. The faculty rate the student's performance daily as satisfactory or unsatisfactory, using predetermined criteria.
Scoring	A satisfactory or unsatisfactory rating for each behavioral item is completed daily. A rating of satisfactory (S) or unsatisfactory (U) for the clinical grade is based on the number of satisfactory and unsatisfactory clinical days, which is predetermined by the faculty. Students must receive an S in the clinical part to pass the course.
Contact Person	Elizabeth Koontz Program Head for Nursing Piedmont Virginia Community College Route 6, Box 1A Charlottesville, VA 22901 (804) 977-3900

Author	**Quinsigamond Community College**
Title	**Clinical Performance Evaluation**
Purpose	To evaluate the student's performance at the freshman level.
Description	A five-page form listing behaviors related to the objectives of the course. Columns for rating the behaviors as satisfactory or unsatisfactory and for remarks are beside each item. The remarks column may be used for anecdotal notes or summaries. The last page is for comments, signatures, and dates of the formal evaluation conference times.
Conceptual Basis	The nursing process.
Administration	Both the student and the instructor complete the tool and share their evaluations at conferences held twice during the first semester, at the midterm, and at the end of the clinical rotation.
Scoring	Starred items are critical behaviors and must be passed satisfactorily to pass the clinical part. If a student receives a U (unsatisfactory) in a behavior, the team meets to evaluate the student's past perfomance to determine whether it is possible to make up the work. If a student receives a U for the clinical part and fails theory, or vice versa, he or she may reapply for admission.
Contact Person	Margaret Barry Coordinator, Nurse Education Program Quinsigamond Community College 670 West Boylston Street Worcester, MA 01606 (617) 853-2300, ext. 273

Author	**Riverside Community College**
Title	**Objective Assessment of Clinical Competence**
Purpose	To evaluate the student's clinical performance.
Description	One-page forms that list critical elements in the care of patients with specific equipment. There are columns beside each element for the instructor to check yes or no Space for comments, signatures, and the final grade is also on the front of the form. These rating tools are used in all semesters and are leveled according to the course.
Administration	The faculty member rates, comments, and signs the form. The student arranges for mastery testing with an instructor. The student is required to be tested in two to three areas each semester. This tool becomes a part of the other clinical evaluation tool, according to the course level.
Scoring	Checks are placed in either a yes or no column, and a final pass/fail grade is given. The test may be repeated until mastery is achieved.
Contact Person	Sharon Evans Dean Allied Health Riverside Community College 4800 Magnolia Riverside, CA 97506 (714) 684-3240

Author	**Rockland Community College, Associate Degree Nursing Program**
Title	**Level-Based Clinical Evaluation Tools**
Purpose	To evaluate the student's clinical performance.
Description	Evaluation tools that contain a list of expected behaviors of students, organized under 10 program objectives. A column to the right of the behaviors is for recording the instructor's comments. The cover sheet for each tool lists the 10 program objectives with columns to the right for the student's and faculty member's evaluations on a satisfactory/unsatisfactory (S/U) basis. Space also is provided for recording the results of tests throughout the term.
Administration	The tool is used throughout the term to record progress and to tally a final evaluation for each course.
Scoring	Performance is assessed as satisfactory or unsatisfactory. Students must satisfactorily meet all objectives to pass the course.
Contact Person	Dr. Frances Marahan Director of Nursing Rockland Community College 145 College Road Suffern, NY 10901 (914) 356-4650

Author	**St. Petersburg Junior College**
Titles	**Clinical Evaluation Basic Nursing Therapy** and **Medical-Surgical Freshman**
Purpose	To evaluate how freshman students apply clinical objectives from the clinical activities package (CAP).
Description	These two tools are used in the freshman year. The first page is an explanation of the evaluation process and general clinical guidelines (professional behavior). The remaining seven to eight pages describe the clinical behaviors to be met and have columns for rating performance and space for comments on each page. The clinical behaviors are organized under the steps of the nursing process. The last page is for a summative narrative, final grades, and signatures.
Conceptual Basis	The nursing process.
Administration	The student completes the tool as a self-evaluation and brings it to the final conference. The instructor completes the tool and has a conference with the student at the end of each eight-week rotation. The instructor keeps anecdotal records to validate the final evaluation. Both sign the evaluation, the student making comments as desired. In this program, the student purchases learning-instruction packages at the beginning of the course. The student is evaluated on the application of clinical objectives from the CAP—a week-by-week package on the clinical focus for the week and is related to the theory and skills being taught. A list of clinical activities and pre- and postconference topics are identified. The student is thereby given direction without direct contact with the faculty member. The tool also provides consistency among faculty members for an entire group of students. Students are also evaluated on the criteria and objectives from the Skills Learning Instructional Package. Each unit of study has only the essential cognitive skills that are necessary for the student to perform the skill.
Scoring	The scoring scale is S (satisfactory), U (unsatisfactory), NA (not applicable), and

NO (not observed). The student must perform satisfactorily on 80 percent of the activities listed and 100 percent on the critical areas marked with an asterisk. If the clinical part is unsatisfactory, the student fails the course but may repeat it as soon as possible.

Contact Person Jodi Parks
Director, Division of Nursing
St. Petersburg Junior College
Box 13489
St. Petersburg, FL 33733
(813) 341-3640

Author	**Trinity Valley Community College**
Title	**Criteria for Teaching Care Plans**
Purpose	To evaluate a teaching care plan.
Description	A one-page, two-sided form with criteria identified for use in writing a teaching care plan. The criteria are organized under nursing-process headings and one "other" category. A three-scale checklist for rating each item is at the left of the page.
Administration	The faculty rates the tool, which is completed for each assignment.
Scoring	Three scales are used: S (satisfactory), NI (needs improvement), and U (unsatisfactory). These scores feed into the clinical grade.
Contact Person	Mary Hardy Trinity Valley Community College 800 Highway 243 West Kaufman, TX 75142 (214) 932-4309

Author	**Waubonsee Community College**
Title	**Psychiatric Nursing Clinical Evaluation**
Purpose	To evaluate the student's clinical performance in a psychiatric nursing course.
Description	A six-page form on which nine main objectives and many specific behaviors are identified for clinical performance. Columns for rating each behavior on a two-point scale are next to the items, as is space for the instructor to record the student's strengths and weaknesses. Ratings are done at the midterm and the final. A page is available for summary evaluations at the midterm and the final and for signatures and the student's comments. The main objectives on this tool are the same as those identified in a course description. Although this was the only tool sent, other tools in this program are constructed similarly.
Administration	The student has a midterm and a final evaluation conference with the instructor. The student is responsible for documenting his or her performance. The instructor rates the student's performance and makes additional comments.
Scoring	At the midterm evaluation, the student's performance is rated as S (satisfactory) or NI (needs improvement). At the final evaluation, the student is rated S or UNS (unsatisfactory). Theory and clinical work are one grade. A U means failure of the course. A student may repeat one time and one course only.
Contact Person	Dr. Helen Baker Director Waubonsee Community College Route 47 at Harter Road Sugar Grove, IL 60554 (312) 466-4811

Author	**Weber State College, Associate Degree Nursing Program**
Titles	**Freshman Evaluation** and **Sophomore Evaluation**
Purpose	To evaluate the student's clinical performance.
Description	These two tools contain four to five pages in which performance objectives are identified under seven headings: assessment, nursing diagnosis, planning, implementation, evaluation, communication, and professional role. Columns are provided to record satisfactory performance (S), needs improvement (N), or academic warning (A) at the midterm and passing performance (P) or failing performance (F) at the end of the term. Space is provided for comments at each designated point of the evaluation, for a final summary statement, and for the instructor's and student's signatures.
Conceptual Basis	The nursing process, communication, and professional role.
Administration	Tools are utilized formatively at the midterm and summatively at the end of the course.
Scoring	Students are rated as S, N, or A at the midterm and as P or F at the end of the term. The student must receive P in all the performance objectives to pass the clinical portion of each course.
Contact Person	Dr. Gerry Hansen Director Nursing Program Weber State College 3750 Harrison Boulevard Ogden, UT 84403 (801) 626-6132

3 Tools for Measuring Affective Outcomes in Associate Degree Nursing Programs

Lois H. Neuman and Carl H. Miller

This chapter provides a representative collection of measurement tools being utilized by associate degree nurse educators to measure affective outcomes in nursing students. Affective outcomes are defined as personal qualities, values, and satisfactions. Tools included in this section are students' evaluations of programs, courses, faculty, and resources; surveys of graduates and employers; students' self-evaluations; and personality assessments.

Author	**Bacone College**
Title	**Survey of Graduates**
Purpose	To determine the need for an accelerated associate degree nursing program specifically for licensed practical nurses.
Description	Three one-page forms asking a series of questions about the curriculum and employment status of the graduate.
Administration	The survey and a self-addressed envelope are mailed to each graduating class. There is no specified date for the mailing.
Scoring	The results are hand-tabulated and written into minutes. They are discussed at a special meeting for evaluating the program.
Contact Person	Billie Tower Chairperson Division of Health Science Bacone College Muskogee, OK 74401 (918) 683-4581

Author	Belmont College
Title	Graduate Questionnaire/Employer Questionnaire
Purpose	To assist in evaluating the Associate Degree Nursing Program.
Description	A one-page form with seven areas related to the adequacy of classroom teaching, the nursing campus laboratory, clinical nursing experiences, decision-making skills, orientation to actual practice, continuing education, and legal/ethical issues to be rated using a five-point scale, ranging from needs improvement (1) to excellent (5). A check is made in the appropriate column.
Conceptual Basis	Roy's adaptation model.
Administration	Sent every two years to associate degree graduates; the employer survey is sent at the same time. Responses are tabulated and reports are made to appropriate college staff to identify the strengths and weaknesses of the program.
Scoring	The rating scale ranges from needs improvement = 1 to excellent = 5
Contact Person	Dr. Anna Hite Dean Belmont College 1900 Belmont Boulevard Nashville, TN 37203 (615) 385-6436

Affective Outcomes

Author	Cecil Community College
Title	**Evaluation of the Neuman Systems Model**
Purpose	To evaluate the Neuman systems model as a basis for developing the curriculum.
Description	An 8-page questionnaire on which graduates of the program respond to statements by circling the adverb that best describes their understanding of the concept. Section 1 addresses concepts of the Neuman model with 40 first-person statements listed under various categories of perception. In Section 2—application of the model—47 third-person items are categorized under the 5 role functions of the nurse.
Conceptual Basis	Neuman systems model.
Administration	Administered to undergraduates of the associate degree nursing program three weeks before and six months after graduation. A longitudinal study is under way, with the results used for revising the curriculum.
Scoring	A 5-level scale of never, rarely, sometimes, mostly, and always.
Contact Person	Lois Lowry Director of Nursing Cecil Community College Associate Degree Nursing Program 1000 North East Road North East, MD 21901 (301) 287-6060

Author	**Central Carolina Community College, Associate Degree Nursing Program**
Title	**Checklist for the Essential Knowledge and Skills of the Beginning RN in the Hospital Setting**
Purpose	To evaluate the Associate Degree Nursing Program.
Description	A 15-page evaluation tool containing 62 items listed under 4 categories: care provider, teacher, manager, and member of a profession; and 8 pages listing psychomotor skills. Graduates are asked to check yes or no for each item. Space is available for suggestions when no is checked.
Administration	Administered after graduation.
Scoring	Each item is scored yes or no according to the following criteria: *Yes* indicates that the graduate possessed the knowledge or ability to perform the behavior at the initial employment. *No* indicates the knowledge or ability was lacking. When no is checked, suggestions are requested.
Contact Person	Gloria H. Peele Nursing Program Central Carolina Community College 530 Carthage Street Sanford, NC 27330 (919) 774-9516

Author	**Charles Stewart Mott Community College**
Title	**Questionnaire for Employers of Mott Community College Associate Degree Nursing Graduates**
Purpose	To help the school understand how employers view the education received by graduates.
Description	This is a five-page tool adapted according to the specific program. General questions are asked about the general utilization and long-range use of associate degree nurses. Specific behaviors are also listed for rating on a five-point rating scale, from very good to not applicable.
Administration	The form is sent to employers. The results are tabulated by a secretary and then reviewed in appropriate committees.
Scoring	Five scales are used: A = very good, B = good, C = average, D = poor, and E = not applicable.
Contact Person	Anita Daus Chairperson Charles Stewart Mott Community College Division of Nursing and Allied Health 1401 East Court Street Flint, MI 48502 (313) 762-0317

Author	**CHRV College of Health Services**
Title	**Evaluation Form for New Graduates**
Purpose	To conduct a postgraduate survey of graduates of the Associate Degree Nursing Program.
Description	The survey has four sections. The first section has 15 objectives of the program with a five-point rating scale for identifying the level of competency. The second section on professional life requests information about professional organizations, journals, and service to the profession. The third section requests information about continuing education, and the fourth section requests demographic data—employment and NCLEX review courses.
Administration	The survey is sent to all new graduates one year after graduation. Directions request graduates to respond by rating items, listing information, selecting between two options, or providing specific responses, as appropriate to the specific questions.
Scoring	The scale for the level of competency (for meeting the objectives of the program) is 5 = excellent, 4 = above average, 3 = average, 2 = below average, and 1 = poor. The results are utilized for informal discussions by the faculty of the findings. As more classes graduate, further data analysis is anticipated.
Contact Person	Carol H. Trent Director CHRV College of Health Services PO Box 1751 Roanoke, VA 24008 (703) 985-8260

Author	**Cochise College**
Title	**Graduate Assessment Form**
Purpose	To evaluate graduates' performance of selected behaviors.
Description	A form with 15 nursing behaviors listed and rated on a 3-point scale and not observed.
Administration	The form is mailed to the employer of each graduate to rate the graduate's performance. A stamped self-addressed envelope is included for returning the form.
Scoring	The rater is asked to check if the graduate performs better, the same, or at a lower level than most graduates with comparable education and experience and if the graduate has or has not been observed in this area.
Contact Person	Dr. Sarah Stark Division Chair Cochise College Douglas, AZ 85607 (602) 364-7943, ext. 216

Author	**Darton College (formerly Albany Junior College) Associate Degree Nursing Program**
Title	**Graduate Survey**
Purpose	To conduct a follow-up of graduates within a year of graduation.
Description	A five-page evaluation tool containing four sections: review time for NCLEX, prepartion time for NCLEX (in specific areas and how well-prepared the graduate felt), clinical experiences, (rating of various clinical experiences) and general (what the school could do to prepare students better for employment and the NCLEX.) Space is provided for any additional comments the graduate may wish to make. A signature is optional.
Administration	The tool is sent to graduates within a year after graduation.
Scoring	Individual data are reported annually in the aggregate.
Contact Person	Betty Ann Page Chairperson Nursing Program Darton College 2400 Gillionville Road Albany, GA 31707 (912) 888-8820

Author	**Darton College (formerly Albany Junior College) Associate Degree Nursing Program**
Title	**Health Care Facility Evaluation of AD Graduate Nursing**
Purpose	To conduct a one-year follow-up of graduates' employers.
Description	A two-page evaluation tool containing three sections: demographic information, management and professional behaviors to be rated on a four-point scale (excellent, good, fair, or needs improvement), and psychomotor skills to be rated on a three-point scale (performs well, performs adequately, or needs improvement). Space is provided for additional comments.
Administration	The tool is sent to graduate employers within a year after graduation.
Scoring	Individual data related to professional behaviors and psychomotor skills are reported annually in the aggregate.
Contact Person	Betty Ann Page Chairperson Nursing Program Darton College 2400 Gillionville Road Albany, GA 31707 (912) 888-8820

Author	**Eastern Oklahoma State College**
Title	**Program Evaluation**
Purpose	To evaluate the nursing program.
Description	A one-page, five-point-scale checklist on which the respondents rate the outcome behaviors by circling the number corresponding to the adverb that best describes their perception. A small space is provided for comments.
Administration	The students complete the checklist, and the faculty uses the information for decision making.
Scoring	A five-point scale of (1) exceptionally well, (2) well, (3) safely, (4) uncertain, and (5) not at all. Scoring is done manually, and a summary is written.
Contact Person	Marsha Green Director of Nursing Education Eastern Oklahoma State College 1301 West Main Wilburton, OK 74578 (918) 465-2361

Author	**Indian River Community College**
Title	**Follow-up Survey of Graduates of the Nursing Programs**
Purpose	To conduct a follow-up survey of graduates of the nursing program to help evaluate the nursing program.
Description	A one-page form asking general questions about the graduates' present employment and evaluation of the nursing program. Space is provided for written suggestions.
Conceptual Basis	Orem's theory of nursing.
Administration	The questionnaire is sent six months after graduation and returned to the coordinator of nursing. After tabulation, it is reviewed by the curriculum committee.
Contact Person	Dr. Erma Kraft Coordinator Indian River Community College 3209 Virginia Avenue Fort Pierce, FL 33454-9003 (407) 468-4778

Author	**Junior College of Albany, Associate Degree Nursing Program**
Title	**Course Evaluation**
Purpose	For students to evaluate courses.
Description	A one-page evaluation form that requests students to comment on classroom experiences, the content of courses, the college laboratory performance test, clinical experiences, and textbooks. Comments must be specific and brief, since there is only a small space for each area.
Administration	Completed by all students at the end of the term.
Scoring	Responses from each student become part of the aggregate data supplied by the total group of students. Data are synthesized and the findings are analyzed.
Contact Person	Joan Maguire Chairperson Nursing Program Junior College of Albany 140 New Scotland Avenue Albany, NY 12205 (518) 445-1734

Author	**Kaskaskia College**
Title	**Employer Follow-up Questionnaire**
Purpose	To evaluate how well graduates are prepared to function as beginning associate degree nurses.
Description	List of behaviors with a five-point rating scale.
Administration	Employers rate the graduates named using the rating scale with 5 as the highest rating.
Scoring	The total is calculated and converted to percentages; then the faculty members examine the results and make changes in the program based on the results.
Contact Person	Violet Draper Director Associate Degree Nursing Program Kaskaskia College Shattuc Road Centralia, IL 62801 (618) 532-1981

Author	**Kaskaskia College**
Title	**Student Self-Evaluation**
Purpose	For students to conduct self-assessments of their progress.
Description	A one-page form listing seven items related to the course about which students are asked to give their opinions. Items include meeting course objectives, progressing satisfactorily with new knowledge gained, improving clinical performance, learning something new about professional behavior, being able to apply theory to clinical, and identifying strengths. Space is provided to list strengths and areas for improvement.
Administration	Student completes the form at the end of the course. The response is kept while the student is in the program and then destroyed when the student graduates.
Scoring	A four-level rating scale is used: strongly agree (SA), agree (A), disagree (D), and strongly disagree (SD). Comments and information about strengths and areas for improvement are tabulated.
Contact Person	Violet Draper Director Associate Degree Nursing Program Kaskaskia College Shattuc Road Centralia, IL 62801 (618) 532-1981

Author	**Mitchell Community College**
Title	**Program Evaluation**
Purpose	To evaluate the student's satisfaction with the nursing program.
Description	A three-page form with statements about the program organized under five headings: administration, faculty, students, curriculum, and facilities. Each item is to be rated on a five-point scale by circling the number that best corresponds to the appropriate word. A space for making suggestions is at the end of the form.
Administration	Graduating students and faculty complete the tool each May at the end of a leadership course, which is the last course in the program. The results are looked at as a whole for any glaring deficits. The curriculum is then revised, if necessary.
Scoring	A five-point scale, 1 (strongly agree) to 5 (strongly disagree), is used. The results are hand-tabulated.
Contact Person	Irene Henline Director Mitchell Community College West Broad Street Statesville, NC 28677 (704) 878-3200

Author	**North Arkansas Community College**
Title	**Course Evaluation**
Purpose	To evaluate the student's satisfaction with a course.
Description	A 3-page form on which there are 33 statements about a course or an instructor.
Administration	The tool is given at the end of each course. The student rates each statement on a rating scale of 1–5. The tool is being revised by the nursing department.
Scoring	A five-point numerical scale is used for rating. The results are used within the department.
Contact Person	Beth Taverner Director North Arkansas Community College Harrison, AR 72601 (501) 743-3000

Author	**Quinsigamond Community College**
Title	**Graduate Survey**
Purpose	For graduates to evaluate the terminal objectives of the program.
Description	An in-house professionally printed 4-page form with 23 general questions and 37 behavioral items to be rated by 2 scales—preparation and utilization. The behaviors relate to the terminal objectives of the program.
Administration	The questionnaire is sent to graduates one year after graduation.
Scoring	The results are tabulated in the registrar's office and then returned to the appropriate committee.
Contact Person	Margaret Barry Coordinator, Nurse Education Program Quinsigamond Community College 670 West Boylston Street Worcester, MA 01606 (617) 853-2300, ext. 273

Author	**San Antonio College**
Title	**Student Clinical Agencies Evaluation Form**
Purpose	To evaluate student's ratings of the clinical agency.
Description	A one-page checklist on which the student rates three areas using a five-point scale. Areas to be rated include atmosphere of the clinical setting, physical environment, and types of assignments. Comments may be written on the form.
Administration	The student completes the checklist at the end of each rotation/semester.
Scoring	A five-point scale is used: always, usually, seldom, never, not apply. Data are analyzed and summarized by computer. The results are used to help faculty make decisions and to share information with the clinical facility regarding the student's rating of the facility.
Contact Person	Dr. Hector Hugo Gonzalez Chairperson San Antonio College 1300 San Pedro Avenue San Antonio, TX 78284 (512) 733-2365

Author	**Southern College of Seventh-Day Adventists, Division of Nursing**
Title	**Evaluation Tool for Clinical Facilities and Agencies**
Purpose	To evaluate clinical facilities.
Description	A two-page evaluation tool that identifies faculty-generated data regarding clinical facilities in the following categories: nursing service, number of personnel by the titles of their positions, other educational programs utilizing the same clinical space, written application of the nursing process, availability of references, physical plant, staffing, and attitude toward students.
Administration	The form is completed by the faculty of courses that use the clinical facility.
Scoring	Short-answer and yes/no responses are required. The results are used for future planning.
Contact Person	Katie Lamb Chairperson Division of Nursing Southern College of Seventh-Day Adventists Collegedale, TN 37315 (615) 238-2942

Author	**Trinity Valley Community College**
Title	**Course Evaluation**
Purpose	To provide feedback on clinical facilities and textbooks used for each course.
Description	A five-page questionnaire on which a student responds to statements about a course using a four-point scale from A to D. The questions are related to objectives, content, instructors, texts, clinical facility, the skills lab, and support services. Written comments are to be made on a blank page.
Administration	At the end of each course, the student completes the tool using a Scantron and may also used the attached blank sheet for written responses.
Scoring	A four-level scale is used: A = excellent, B = good, C = fair, and D = poor. The results are tabulated by Scantron and shared in individual faculty meetings and in curriculum committees. Changes have been made in the placement of students, textbooks, and so forth.
Contact Person	Mary Hardy Trinity Valley Community College 800 Highway 243 West Kaufman, TX 75142 (214) 932-4309

Author	**Weber State College, Associate Degree Nursing Program**
Title	**"I Made the Difference" Preceptor Program**
Purpose	To obtain student's self-assessments of the preceptor experience.
Description	A two-page form on which a student records a particular incident, describes it in detail, and evaluates it in light of how his or her nursing action made a difference to the patient.
Administration	The student completes the form at the conclusion of the preceptorship experience.
Scoring	The tool is used to give the student the opportunity to assess the value of the preceptorship experience. The assessment does not influence the student's grade for the course.
Contact Person	Dr. Gerry Hansen Director Nursing Program Weber State College 3750 Harrison Boulevard Ogden, UT 84403 (801) 626-6132

Suggested References on Reliability and Validity

Berk, R.A. (Ed.). (1980) *Criterion-referenced measurement: The state of the art*. Baltimore, MD: Johns Hopkins University Press.

Polit, D.F. and Hungler, B. P. (1987). *Nursing research principles and methods* (3rd ed.). Philadelphia: J. B. Lippincott.

Thorndike, R. L. and Hagen, E. (1977) *Measurement and evaluation in psychology and education* (4th ed.). New York: John Wiley & Sons.

Waltz, C. F., Strickland, O. L., and Lenz, E. R. (1984). *Measurement in nursing research*. Philadelphia: F. A. Davis.

DATE DUE			
MAR 2 2 1992			
MAR 2 6 1992			
GAYLORD			PRINTED IN U.S.A.